DIABETIC TYPE 1 VEGETARIAN COOKBOOK FOR BEGINNERS

Explore the Flavors of Plant-Based Cooking with Essential Recipes, Nutrition Insights, and Meal Planning Strategies to Thrive with Type 1 Diabetes, Perfect for Newbies to Vegetarian Cuisine

T. John

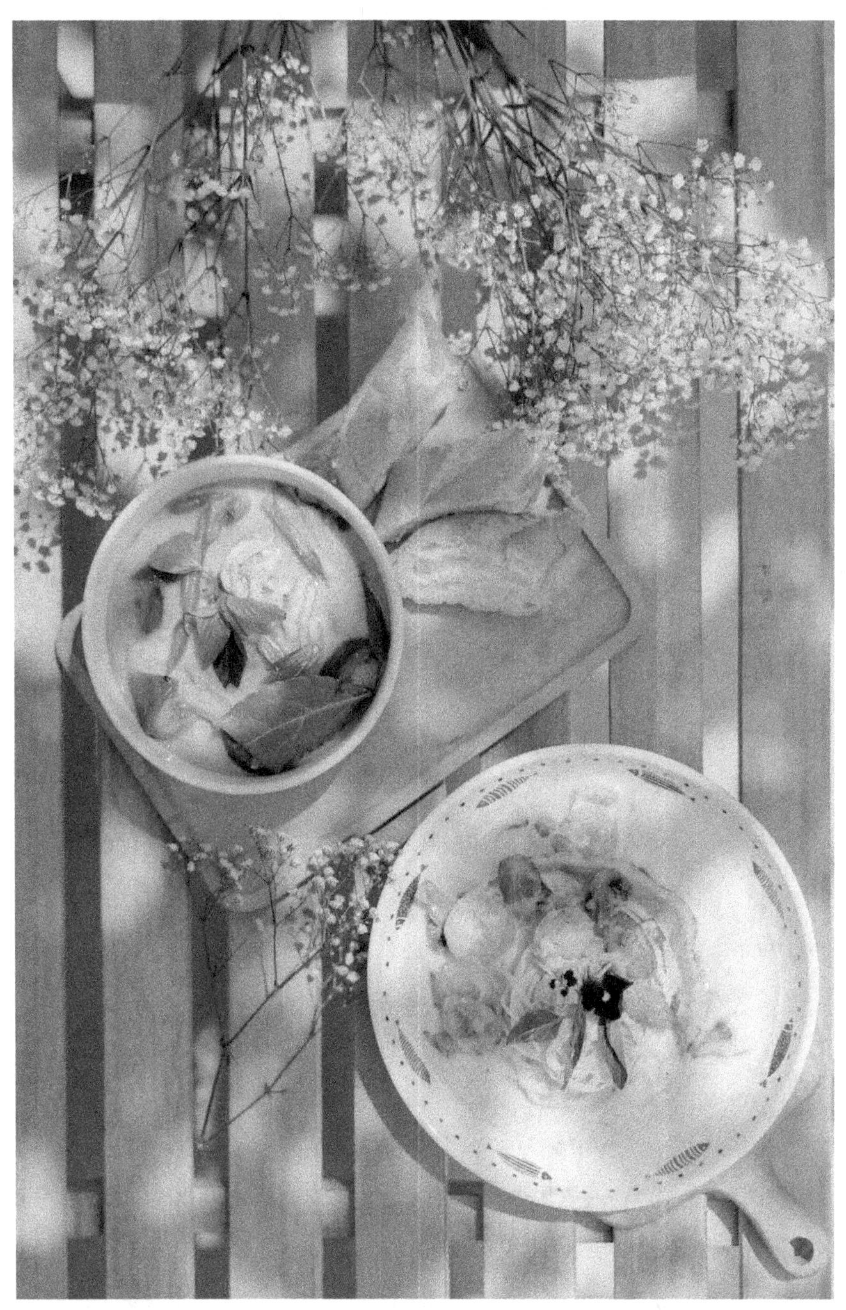

TABLE OF CONTENTS

INTRODUCTION 9

Understanding Type 1 Diabetes: 9

Diet: Your Co-Pilot in Blood Sugar Management 10

Can a Vegetarian Diet Benefit Your Diabetic Journey? 10

Essential Tips for Vegetarian Beginners with Type 1 Diabetes 11

Chapter 1: 30 Day Meal Plan 13

Week 1: 13

Week 2: 15

Week 3: 17

Week 4: 19

Chapter 2: Breakfast Recipes 23

Avocado Toast with Cherry Tomatoes.............................. 23

Greek Yogurt with Berries and Chia Seeds 24

Spinach and Mushroom Omelette 25

Almond Flour Pancakes 26

Tofu Scramble with Veggies...................................... 27

Quinoa Breakfast Bowl 28

Cinnamon Apple Oatmeal.. 29

Smoothie Bowl with Nuts and Seeds 30

Chia Pudding with Almond Milk 31

Baked Sweet Potato with Cinnamon 32

Veggie Breakfast Burrito 33

Peanut Butter Banana Smoothie... 34

Veggie Frittata... 35

Whole Wheat Bagel with Cream Cheese and Tomato 36

Overnight Oats with Blueberries 37

Chapter 3: Lunch Recipes.. 39

Lentil and Vegetable Soup 39

Chickpea Salad Sandwich 40

Quinoa and Black Bean Salad 42

Spinach and Feta Stuffed Peppers 43

Tomato Basil Soup 44

Tofu and Veggie Stir-Fry 45

Mediterranean Veggie Wrap 46

Cauliflower Rice Burrito Bowl 47

Zucchini Noodles with Pesto.. 49

Caprese Salad with Balsamic Glaze 50

Grilled Portobello Mushroom Burger 51

Sweet Potato and Black Bean Tacos 52

Kale and Quinoa Salad.. 53

Hummus and Veggie Wrap 54

Vegetable Paella 55

Chapter 4: Dinner Recipes 57

Eggplant Parmesan.. 57

Stuffed Bell Peppers.. 58

Spaghetti Squash with Marinara Sauce 60

Veggie Stir-Fry with Tofu.. 61

Cauliflower Crust Pizza 63

Mushroom and Spinach Lasagna 64

Sweet Potato and Lentil Curry 66

Baked Ziti with Vegetables 67

Stuffed Acorn Squash.. 69

Ratatouille 71

Broccoli and Cheddar Stuffed Potatoes 72

Vegetable Korma.. 73

Black Bean and Corn Enchiladas 75

Grilled Vegetable Skewers 77

Chickpea and Spinach Stew 78

Chapter 5: Snacks and Appetizers 80

Hummus with Veggie Sticks.. 80

Baked Kale Chips.. 81

Roasted Chickpeas 82

Guacamole with Whole Grain Crackers.. 83

Veggie Spring Rolls 84

Greek Yogurt Dip with Cucumber Slices 85

Stuffed Mini Peppers.. 86

Almond Butter Apple Slices 87

Edamame with Sea Salt.. 88

Spicy Roasted Cauliflower Bites.. 89

Caprese Skewers 90

Veggie Sushi Rolls.. 91

Parmesan Zucchini Fries 92

Mini Quiche Cups 93

Berry and Nut Mix 94

Chapter 6: Desserts 96

Chia Seed Pudding with Mango................................ 96

Chocolate Avocado Mousse.................................... 97

Baked Apples with Cinnamon................................... 98

Greek Yogurt Parfait with Berries 99

Almond Flour Brownies...................................... 100

Banana Ice Cream 101

Carrot Cake Energy Balls................................... 102

Strawberry Chia Jam Bars.................................. 103

Apple Cinnamon Muffins.................................... 104

Blueberry Crumble... 105

Coconut Macaroons.. 106

Dark Chocolate Covered Almonds 107

Pumpkin Pie Bites... 107

Lemon Yogurt Popsicles 108

Mixed Berry Sorbet.. 109

Chapter 7: Smoothies 111

Green Detox Smoothie...................................... 111

Berry Blast Smoothie 112

Tropical Mango Smoothie................................... 113

Spinach and Avocado Smoothie 114

Peanut Butter Banana Smoothie............................ 115

Chocolate Protein Smoothie................................ 116

Pineapple Kale Smoothie 117

Beetroot and Berry Smoothie............................... 118

Carrot Ginger Smoothie 119

Apple Pie Smoothie.. 120

Citrus Sunshine Smoothie 121

Strawberry Banana Smoothie.. 122

Matcha Green Tea Smoothie.. 123

Watermelon Mint Smoothie 124

Chia Seed Power Smoothie 125

CONCLUSION **126**

INTRODUCTION

I magine your body is a complex spaceship, and blood sugar is its fuel. In type 1 diabetes, the pancreas malfunctions, leaving the ship without its internal fuel regulator. This is where you, the captain, step in. You become responsible for managing the spaceship's fuel levels through a combination of insulin injections and strategic dietary choices. Understanding type 1 diabetes, its dietary connection, and how a vegetarian diet can fit in empowers you to navigate this journey.

Understanding Type 1 Diabetes:

Type 1 diabetes is an autoimmune disease where the body attacks the insulin-producing cells in the pancreas. Insulin acts like a key, unlocking the door for glucose (sugar) from your bloodstream to enter your cells and provide energy. Without enough insulin, the fuel gauge malfunctions. Excess sugar builds up in your bloodstream, leading to a variety of health issues.

Diet: Your Co-Pilot in Blood Sugar Management

The foods you eat directly impact your blood sugar levels. Carbohydrates, found in grains, fruits, and vegetables, are broken down into glucose. This is why dietary management is crucial for people with type 1 diabetes. By carefully planning meals and understanding how different foods affect your blood sugar, you can work alongside your insulin to maintain optimal fuel levels for your spaceship.

Can a Vegetarian Diet Benefit Your Diabetic Journey?

A well-planned vegetarian diet can be a fantastic co-pilot for managing type 1 diabetes. Here's why:

- **Fiber Power:** Vegetarian diets are naturally rich in fiber, found in vegetables, fruits, and legumes. Fiber slows down the absorption of glucose into your bloodstream, leading to steadier blood sugar levels.
- **Weight Management:** Vegetarian diets tend to be lower in calories and saturated fat, which can aid in weight management. Maintaining a healthy weight can significantly improve blood sugar control.

- **Nutrient Richness:** A vegetarian diet packed with colorful vegetables ensures a good intake of vitamins, minerals, and antioxidants, all vital for overall health and disease prevention.

Essential Tips for Vegetarian Beginners with Type 1 Diabetes

- **Embrace Protein Powerhouses:** Include protein sources like lentils, beans, tofu, and tempeh in your meals to keep you feeling full and provide sustained energy.
- **Carb Counting is Key:** Learn to count carbohydrates and factor them into your insulin dosing plan. This helps you anticipate blood sugar spikes.
- **Don't Fear Healthy Fats**: Include healthy fats like nuts, seeds, and avocado in moderation to promote satiety and aid in nutrient absorption.
- **Read Labels Like a Pro**: Pay close attention to hidden sugars in processed vegetarian foods. Choose whole foods whenever possible.

Remember, a vegetarian diet for type 1 diabetes is a journey, not a destination. Experiment with different recipes, find a support group, and celebrate your milestones. With the right knowledge and a healthy dose of self-compassion, you can navigate your diabetic journey with confidence, using a vegetarian diet as your trusty co-pilot.

Chapter 1: 30 Day Meal Plan

Week 1:

Day 1

- Breakfast: Avocado Toast with Cherry Tomatoes
- Lunch: Lentil and Vegetable Soup
- Dinner: Eggplant Parmesan
- Snack: Hummus with Veggie Sticks
- Dessert: Chia Seed Pudding with Mango

Day 2

- Breakfast: Greek Yogurt with Berries and Chia Seeds
- Lunch: Chickpea Salad Sandwich
- Dinner: Stuffed Bell Peppers
- Snack: Baked Kale Chips
- Dessert: Chocolate Avocado Mousse

Day 3

- Breakfast: Spinach and Mushroom Omelette
- Lunch: Quinoa and Black Bean Salad
- Dinner: Spaghetti Squash with Marinara Sauce
- Snack: Roasted Chickpeas
- Dessert: Baked Apples with Cinnamon

Day 4

- Breakfast: Almond Flour Pancakes
- Lunch: Spinach and Feta Stuffed Peppers
- Dinner: Veggie Stir-Fry with Tofu
- Snack: Guacamole with Whole Grain Crackers
- Dessert: Greek Yogurt Parfait with Berries

Day 5

- Breakfast: Tofu Scramble with Veggies
- Lunch: Tomato Basil Soup
- Dinner: Cauliflower Crust Pizza
- Snack: Veggie Spring Rolls
- Dessert: Almond Flour Brownies

Day 6

- Breakfast: Quinoa Breakfast Bowl
- Lunch: Tofu and Veggie Stir-Fry
- Dinner: Mushroom and Spinach Lasagna
- Snack: Greek Yogurt Dip with Cucumber Slices
- Dessert: Banana Ice Cream

Day 7

- Breakfast: Cinnamon Apple Oatmeal
- Lunch: Mediterranean Veggie Wrap

- Dinner: Sweet Potato and Lentil Curry
- Snack: Stuffed Mini Peppers
- Dessert: Carrot Cake Energy Balls

Week 2:

Day 8

- Breakfast: Smoothie Bowl with Nuts and Seeds
- Lunch: Cauliflower Rice Burrito Bowl
- Dinner: Baked Ziti with Vegetables
- Snack: Almond Butter Apple Slices
- Dessert: Strawberry Chia Jam Bars

Day 9

- Breakfast: Chia Pudding with Almond Milk
- Lunch: Zucchini Noodles with Pesto
- Dinner: Stuffed Acorn Squash
- Snack: Edamame with Sea Salt
- Dessert: Apple Cinnamon Muffins

Day 10

- Breakfast: Baked Sweet Potato with Cinnamon
- Lunch: Caprese Salad with Balsamic Glaze
- Dinner: Ratatouille

- Snack: Spicy Roasted Cauliflower Bites
- Dessert: Blueberry Crumble

Day 11

- Breakfast: Veggie Breakfast Burrito
- Lunch: Grilled Portobello Mushroom Burger
- Dinner: Broccoli and Cheddar Stuffed Potatoes
- Snack: Caprese Skewers
- Dessert: Coconut Macaroons

Day 12

- Breakfast: Peanut Butter Banana Smoothie
- Lunch: Sweet Potato and Black Bean Tacos
- Dinner: Vegetable Korma
- Snack: Veggie Sushi Rolls
- Dessert: Dark Chocolate Covered Almonds

Day 13

- Breakfast: Veggie Frittata
- Lunch: Kale and Quinoa Salad
- Dinner: Black Bean and Corn Enchiladas
- Snack: Parmesan Zucchini Fries
- Dessert: Pumpkin Pie Bites

Day 14

- Breakfast: Whole Wheat Bagel with Cream Cheese and Tomato
- Lunch: Hummus and Veggie Wrap
- Dinner: Grilled Vegetable Skewers
- Snack: Mini Quiche Cups
- Dessert: Lemon Yogurt Popsicles

Week 3:

Day 15

- Breakfast: Overnight Oats with Blueberries
- Lunch: Vegetable Paella
- Dinner: Chickpea and Spinach Stew
- Snack: Berry and Nut Mix
- Dessert: Mixed Berry Sorbet

Day 16

- Breakfast: Avocado Toast with Cherry Tomatoes
- Lunch: Lentil and Vegetable Soup
- Dinner: Eggplant Parmesan
- Snack: Hummus with Veggie Sticks
- Dessert: Chia Seed Pudding with Mango

Day 17

- Breakfast: Greek Yogurt with Berries and Chia Seeds
- Lunch: Chickpea Salad Sandwich
- Dinner: Stuffed Bell Peppers
- Snack: Baked Kale Chips
- Dessert: Chocolate Avocado Mousse

Day 18

- Breakfast: Spinach and Mushroom Omelette
- Lunch: Quinoa and Black Bean Salad
- Dinner: Spaghetti Squash with Marinara Sauce
- Snack: Roasted Chickpeas
- Dessert: Baked Apples with Cinnamon

Day 19

- Breakfast: Almond Flour Pancakes
- Lunch: Spinach and Feta Stuffed Peppers
- Dinner: Veggie Stir-Fry with Tofu
- Snack: Guacamole with Whole Grain Crackers
- Dessert: Greek Yogurt Parfait with Berries

Day 20

- Breakfast: Tofu Scramble with Veggies
- Lunch: Tomato Basil Soup

- Dinner: Cauliflower Crust Pizza

- Snack: Veggie Spring Rolls

- Dessert: Almond Flour Brownies

Day 21

- Breakfast: Quinoa Breakfast Bowl

- Lunch: Tofu and Veggie Stir-Fry

- Dinner: Mushroom and Spinach Lasagna

- Snack: Greek Yogurt Dip with Cucumber Slices

- Dessert: Banana Ice Cream

Week 4:

Day 22

- Breakfast: Cinnamon Apple Oatmeal

- Lunch: Mediterranean Veggie Wrap

- Dinner: Sweet Potato and Lentil Curry

- Snack: Stuffed Mini Peppers

- Dessert: Carrot Cake Energy Balls

Day 23

- Breakfast: Smoothie Bowl with Nuts and Seeds

- Lunch: Cauliflower Rice Burrito Bowl

- Dinner: Baked Ziti with Vegetables

- Snack: Almond Butter Apple Slices
- Dessert: Strawberry Chia Jam Bars

Day 24

- Breakfast: Chia Pudding with Almond Milk
- Lunch: Zucchini Noodles with Pesto
- Dinner: Stuffed Acorn Squash
- Snack: Edamame with Sea Salt
- Dessert: Apple Cinnamon Muffins

Day 25

- Breakfast: Baked Sweet Potato with Cinnamon
- Lunch: Caprese Salad with Balsamic Glaze
- Dinner: Ratatouille
- Snack: Spicy Roasted Cauliflower Bites
- Dessert: Blueberry Crumble

Day 26

- Breakfast: Veggie Breakfast Burrito
- Lunch: Grilled Portobello Mushroom Burger
- Dinner: Broccoli and Cheddar Stuffed Potatoes
- Snack: Caprese Skewers
- Dessert: Coconut Macaroons

Day 27

- Breakfast: Peanut Butter Banana Smoothie
- Lunch: Sweet Potato and Black Bean Tacos
- Dinner: Vegetable Korma
- Snack: Veggie Sushi Rolls
- Dessert: Dark Chocolate Covered Almonds

Day 28

- Breakfast: Veggie Frittata
- Lunch: Kale and Quinoa Salad
- Dinner: Black Bean and Corn Enchiladas
- Snack: Parmesan Zucchini Fries
- Dessert: Pumpkin Pie Bites

Day 29

- Breakfast: Whole Wheat Bagel with Cream Cheese and Tomato
- Lunch: Hummus and Veggie Wrap
- Dinner: Grilled Vegetable Skewers
- Snack: Mini Quiche Cups
- Dessert: Lemon Yogurt Popsicles

Day 30

- Breakfast: Overnight Oats with Blueberries

- Lunch: Vegetable Paella

- Dinner: Chickpea and Spinach Stew

- Snack: Berry and Nut Mix

- Dessert: Mixed Berry Sorbet

Chapter 2: Breakfast Recipes

Starting your day with a healthy breakfast is especially important for those managing Type 1 Diabetes. This chapter provides a variety of nutritious and delicious vegetarian breakfast recipes that are not only easy to prepare but also balanced to help maintain your blood sugar levels.

Avocado Toast with Cherry Tomatoes

Ingredients:

- 1 slice whole grain bread
- 1/2 avocado
- 5 cherry tomatoes, halved
- Salt and pepper to taste
- 1 tsp lemon juice

Instructions:

1. Toast the bread.
2. Mash the avocado with lemon juice, salt, and pepper.
3. Spread the avocado on the toast and top with cherry tomatoes.

Nutrition Information:

- Calories: 220
- Protein: 5g
- Carbohydrates: 22g
- Fat: 14g
- Fiber: 8g
- Sugar: 2g
- Portion Size: 1 slice

Greek Yogurt with Berries and Chia Seeds

Ingredients:

- 1 cup Greek yogurt
- 1/2 cup mixed berries (blueberries, strawberries, raspberries)
- 1 tbsp chia seeds
- 1 tsp honey (optional)

Instructions:

1. Place the Greek yogurt in a bowl.
2. Top with mixed berries and chia seeds.
3. Drizzle with honey if desired.

Nutrition Information:

- Calories: 200
- Protein: 15g
- Carbohydrates: 20g
- Fat: 6g
- Fiber: 5g
- Sugar: 12g
- Portion Size: 1 bowl

Spinach and Mushroom Omelette

Ingredients:

- 2 eggs
- 1/4 cup spinach, chopped
- 1/4 cup mushrooms, sliced
- 1 tbsp milk
- Salt and pepper to taste
- 1 tsp olive oil

Instructions:

1. Whisk eggs with milk, salt, and pepper.
2. Heat olive oil in a pan and sauté spinach and mushrooms.
3. Pour the egg mixture over the veggies and cook until set.

Nutrition Information:

- Calories: 180
- Protein: 12g
- Carbohydrates: 3g
- Fat: 14g
- Fiber: 1g
- Sugar: 1g
- Portion Size: 1 omelette

Almond Flour Pancakes

Ingredients:

- 1 cup almond flour
- 2 eggs
- 1/4 cup almond milk
- 1 tsp baking powder
- 1 tsp vanilla extract
- 1 tbsp coconut oil

Instructions:

1. Mix almond flour, baking powder, eggs, almond milk, and vanilla extract.
2. Heat coconut oil in a pan.

3. Pour batter into the pan and cook pancakes until golden brown on both sides.

Nutrition Information:

- Calories: 280
- Protein: 10g
- Carbohydrates: 8g
- Fat: 24g
- Fiber: 4g
- Sugar: 2g
- Portion Size: 3 pancakes

Tofu Scramble with Veggies

Ingredients:

- 1/2 block firm tofu, crumbled
- 1/4 cup bell peppers, diced
- 1/4 cup onions, diced
- 1/4 cup spinach, chopped
- 1 tsp turmeric
- Salt and pepper to taste
- 1 tbsp olive oil

Instructions:

1. Heat olive oil in a pan and sauté onions and bell peppers.

2. Add crumbled tofu, spinach, turmeric, salt, and pepper.

3. Cook until veggies are tender and tofu is heated through.

Nutrition Information:

- Calories: 180
- Protein: 12g
- Carbohydrates: 8g
- Fat: 12g
- Fiber: 3g
- Sugar: 2g
- Portion Size: 1 cup

Quinoa Breakfast Bowl

Ingredients:

- 1/2 cup cooked quinoa
- 1/4 cup almond milk
- 1/2 banana, sliced
- 1 tbsp almonds, chopped
- 1 tsp honey

Instructions:

1. Combine quinoa and almond milk in a bowl.
2. Top with banana slices and chopped almonds.
3. Drizzle with honey.

Nutrition Information:

- Calories: 250
- Protein: 6g
- Carbohydrates: 38g
- Fat: 9g
- Fiber: 5g
- Sugar: 12g
- Portion Size: 1 bowl

Cinnamon Apple Oatmeal

Ingredients:

- 1/2 cup rolled oats
- 1 cup water or almond milk
- 1/2 apple, diced
- 1 tsp cinnamon
- 1 tsp honey (optional)

Instructions:

1. Cook oats in water or almond milk as per package instructions.
2. Stir in diced apple and cinnamon.
3. Drizzle with honey if desired.

Nutrition Information:

- Calories: 220
- Protein: 5g
- Carbohydrates: 42g
- Fat: 4g
- Fiber: 6g
- Sugar: 12g
- Portion Size: 1 bowl

Smoothie Bowl with Nuts and Seeds

Ingredients:

- 1 banana
- 1/2 cup frozen berries
- 1/2 cup almond milk
- 1 tbsp chia seeds
- 1 tbsp almonds, sliced

Instructions:

1. Blend banana, berries, and almond milk until smooth.
2. Pour into a bowl and top with chia seeds and almonds.

Nutrition Information:

- Calories: 250
- Protein: 5g
- Carbohydrates: 45g
- Fat: 9g
- Fiber: 8g
- Sugar: 20g
- Portion Size: 1 bowl

Chia Pudding with Almond Milk

Ingredients:

- 1/4 cup chia seeds
- 1 cup almond milk
- 1 tsp vanilla extract
- 1 tsp honey

Instructions:

1. Mix chia seeds, almond milk, vanilla extract, and honey.
2. Refrigerate overnight.

3. Stir before serving.

Nutrition Information:

- Calories: 180
- Protein: 4g
- Carbohydrates: 18g
- Fat: 9g
- Fiber: 10g
- Sugar: 6g
- Portion Size: 1 cup

Baked Sweet Potato with Cinnamon

Ingredients:

- 1 medium sweet potato
- 1 tsp cinnamon
- 1 tsp honey

Instructions:

1. Preheat oven to 400°F (200°C).
2. Bake sweet potato for 45 minutes or until tender.
3. Slice open and sprinkle with cinnamon and honey.

Nutrition Information:

- Calories: 160
- Protein: 2g
- Carbohydrates: 37g
- Fat: 0g
- Fiber: 6g
- Sugar: 12g
- Portion Size: 1 sweet potato

Veggie Breakfast Burrito

Ingredients:

- 1 whole wheat tortilla
- 1/4 cup black beans, cooked
- 1/4 cup bell peppers, diced
- 1/4 cup onions, diced
- 1/4 cup spinach, chopped
- 1 tbsp salsa

Instructions:

1. Sauté bell peppers, onions, and spinach.
2. Fill the tortilla with beans and sautéed veggies.
3. Top with salsa and wrap.

Nutrition Information:

- Calories: 250
- Protein: 10g
- Carbohydrates: 42g
- Fat: 6g
- Fiber: 10g
- Sugar: 4g
- Portion Size: 1 burrito

Peanut Butter Banana Smoothie

Ingredients:

- 1 banana
- 1 cup almond milk
- 1 tbsp peanut butter
- 1 tsp honey
- 1/2 tsp cinnamon

Instructions:

1. Blend all ingredients until smooth.
2. Serve immediately.

Nutrition Information:

- Calories: 250

- Protein: 6g

- Carbohydrates: 35g

- Fat: 11g

- Fiber: 5g

- Sugar: 20g

- Portion Size: 1 smoothie

Veggie Frittata

Ingredients:

- 4 eggs

- 1/4 cup bell peppers, diced

- 1/4 cup zucchini, diced

- 1/4 cup onions, diced

- Salt and pepper to taste

- 1 tbsp olive oil

Instructions:

1. Preheat oven to 375°F (190°C).

2. Sauté veggies in olive oil until tender.

3. Whisk eggs with salt and pepper, pour over veggies, and bake for 20 minutes.

Nutrition Information:

- Calories: 200
- Protein: 12g
- Carbohydrates: 5g
- Fat: 15g
- Fiber: 2g
- Sugar: 3g
- Portion Size: 1 slice

Whole Wheat Bagel with Cream Cheese and Tomato

Ingredients:

- 1 whole wheat bagel
- 2 tbsp cream cheese
- 1 tomato, sliced
- Salt and pepper to taste

Instructions:

1. Toast the bagel.
2. Spread cream cheese on each half.
3. Top with tomato slices, salt, and pepper.

Nutrition Information:

- Calories: 300
- Protein: 10g
- Carbohydrates: 45g
- Fat: 10g
- Fiber: 5g
- Sugar: 6g
- Portion Size: 1 bagel

Overnight Oats with Blueberries

Ingredients:

- 1/2 cup rolled oats
- 1/2 cup almond milk
- 1/4 cup blueberries
- 1 tsp honey
- 1 tsp chia seeds

Instructions:

1. Combine oats, almond milk, blueberries, honey, and chia seeds in a jar.
2. Refrigerate overnight.
3. Stir before serving.

Nutrition Information:

- Calories: 220
- Protein: 6g
- Carbohydrates: 38g
- Fat: 5g
- Fiber: 6g
- Sugar: 12g
- Portion Size: 1 jar

Chapter 3: Lunch Recipes

Creating nutritious and delicious lunch options is essential for maintaining stable blood sugar levels and overall health, especially for individuals with Type 1 diabetes. These vegetarian recipes are designed to be both satisfying and easy to prepare, ensuring you can enjoy a variety of flavors and nutrients without spending too much time in the kitchen.

Lentil and Vegetable Soup

Ingredients:

- 1 cup dried lentils, rinsed
- 1 onion, chopped
- 2 carrots, diced
- 2 celery stalks, diced
- 3 garlic cloves, minced
- 1 can (14.5 oz) diced tomatoes
- 4 cups vegetable broth
- 1 tsp dried thyme
- 1 tsp cumin
- Salt and pepper to taste
- 2 cups spinach, chopped

Instructions:

1. In a large pot, sauté the onion, carrots, celery, and garlic until soft.
2. Add the lentils, diced tomatoes, vegetable broth, thyme, and cumin.
3. Bring to a boil, then reduce heat and simmer for 25-30 minutes.
4. Stir in spinach and cook until wilted.
5. Season with salt and pepper.

Nutrition Information (per serving):

- Calories: 180
- Protein: 10g
- Carbohydrates: 30g
- Fat: 1g
- Fiber: 10g
- Sugar: 6g
- Portion Size: 1 cup

Chickpea Salad Sandwich

Ingredients:

- 1 can (15 oz) chickpeas, drained and mashed
- 1 celery stalk, diced

- 2 tbsp vegan mayonnaise
- 1 tbsp Dijon mustard
- 1 tbsp lemon juice
- Salt and pepper to taste
- 4 slices whole grain bread
- Lettuce leaves
- Tomato slices

Instructions:

1. In a bowl, mix mashed chickpeas, celery, mayonnaise, mustard, lemon juice, salt, and pepper.
2. Spread the chickpea mixture on two slices of bread.
3. Top with lettuce and tomato, then cover with remaining bread slices.

Nutrition Information (per sandwich):

- Calories: 320
- Protein: 12g
- Carbohydrates: 50g
- Fat: 8g
- Fiber: 10g
- Sugar: 4g
- Portion Size: 1 sandwich

Quinoa and Black Bean Salad

Ingredients:

- 1 cup quinoa, cooked
- 1 can (15 oz) black beans, rinsed and drained
- 1 red bell pepper, diced
- 1 avocado, diced
- 1/4 cup red onion, finely chopped
- 1/4 cup cilantro, chopped
- Juice of 1 lime
- 2 tbsp olive oil
- Salt and pepper to taste

Instructions:

1. In a large bowl, combine quinoa, black beans, bell pepper, avocado, red onion, and cilantro.
2. In a small bowl, whisk together lime juice, olive oil, salt, and pepper.
3. Pour dressing over the salad and toss to combine.

Nutrition Information (per serving):

- Calories: 250
- Protein: 8g
- Carbohydrates: 35g
- Fat: 10g

- Fiber: 10g

- Sugar: 2g

- Portion Size: 1 cup

Spinach and Feta Stuffed Peppers

Ingredients:

- 4 bell peppers, halved and seeded

- 2 cups cooked quinoa

- 1 cup spinach, chopped

- 1/2 cup feta cheese, crumbled

- 1/4 cup red onion, chopped

- 1 tsp dried oregano

- Salt and pepper to taste

Instructions:

1. Preheat oven to 375°F (190°C).

2. In a bowl, mix quinoa, spinach, feta, red onion, oregano, salt, and pepper.

3. Stuff each bell pepper half with the quinoa mixture.

4. Place stuffed peppers in a baking dish and bake for 25-30 minutes.

Nutrition Information (per pepper half):

- Calories: 200
- Protein: 7g
- Carbohydrates: 28g
- Fat: 7g
- Fiber: 5g
- Sugar: 5g
- Portion Size: 1 stuffed pepper half

Tomato Basil Soup

Ingredients:

- 1 tbsp olive oil
- 1 onion, chopped
- 3 garlic cloves, minced
- 4 cups tomatoes, chopped
- 2 cups vegetable broth
- 1/4 cup fresh basil, chopped
- Salt and pepper to taste

Instructions:

1. Heat olive oil in a pot over medium heat. Sauté onion and garlic until soft.
2. Add tomatoes and vegetable broth, bring to a boil.

3. Reduce heat and simmer for 20 minutes.

4. Puree the soup with an immersion blender.

5. Stir in fresh basil and season with salt and pepper.

Nutrition Information (per serving):

- Calories: 150

- Protein: 3g

- Carbohydrates: 22g

- Fat: 5g

- Fiber: 4g

- Sugar: 12g

- Portion Size: 1 cup

Tofu and Veggie Stir-Fry

Ingredients:

- 1 block firm tofu, cubed

- 2 tbsp soy sauce

- 1 tbsp sesame oil

- 2 cups mixed vegetables (broccoli, bell pepper, carrots, snap peas)

- 1 tbsp grated ginger

- 2 garlic cloves, minced

- 1 tbsp cornstarch

- 1/4 cup water

Instructions:

1. Marinate tofu in soy sauce for 10 minutes.
2. Heat sesame oil in a pan, add tofu and cook until golden.
3. Add vegetables, ginger, and garlic, stir-fry for 5 minutes.
4. Mix cornstarch and water, pour into the pan and cook until thickened.

Nutrition Information (per serving):

- Calories: 200
- Protein: 15g
- Carbohydrates: 12g
- Fat: 10g
- Fiber: 4g
- Sugar: 3g
- Portion Size: 1 cup

Mediterranean Veggie Wrap

Ingredients:

- 1 whole grain wrap
- 1/4 cup hummus
- 1/4 cup cucumber, sliced

- 1/4 cup tomato, sliced

- 1/4 cup red bell pepper, sliced

- 1/4 cup spinach

- 2 tbsp feta cheese, crumbled

Instructions:

1. Spread hummus on the wrap.

2. Layer cucumber, tomato, bell pepper, spinach, and feta cheese.

3. Roll up the wrap tightly.

Nutrition Information (per wrap):

- Calories: 300

- Protein: 10g

- Carbohydrates: 40g

- Fat: 10g

- Fiber: 8g

- Sugar: 4g

- Portion Size: 1 wrap

Cauliflower Rice Burrito Bowl

Ingredients:

- 2 cups cauliflower rice

- 1 can (15 oz) black beans, rinsed and drained
- 1 avocado, diced
- 1 cup corn kernels
- 1/2 cup salsa
- 1/4 cup cilantro, chopped
- Juice of 1 lime
- Salt and pepper to taste

Instructions:

1. Cook cauliflower rice according to package instructions.
2. In a bowl, combine cauliflower rice, black beans, avocado, corn, salsa, cilantro, and lime juice.
3. Season with salt and pepper.

Nutrition Information (per bowl):

- Calories: 250
- Protein: 8g
- Carbohydrates: 35g
- Fat: 10g
- Fiber: 12g
- Sugar: 5g
- Portion Size: 1 bowl

Zucchini Noodles with Pesto

Ingredients:

- 2 large zucchinis, spiralized
- 1 cup basil leaves
- 1/4 cup pine nuts
- 1/4 cup Parmesan cheese, grated
- 2 garlic cloves
- 1/4 cup olive oil
- Salt and pepper to taste

Instructions:

1. In a food processor, blend basil, pine nuts, Parmesan, garlic, and olive oil until smooth.
2. Toss zucchini noodles with pesto sauce.
3. Season with salt and pepper.

Nutrition Information (per serving):

- Calories: 220
- Protein: 6g
- Carbohydrates: 8g
- Fat: 20g
- Fiber: 3g
- Sugar: 4g
- Portion Size: 1 cup

Caprese Salad with Balsamic Glaze

Ingredients:

- 2 cups cherry tomatoes, halved
- 1 cup fresh mozzarella balls, halved
- 1/4 cup fresh basil leaves
- 2 tbsp balsamic glaze
- 1 tbsp olive oil
- Salt and pepper to taste

Instructions:

1. In a bowl, combine cherry tomatoes, mozzarella, and basil.
2. Drizzle with balsamic glaze and olive oil.
3. Season with salt and pepper.

Nutrition Information (per serving):

- Calories: 180
- Protein: 8g
- Carbohydrates: 10g
- Fat: 12g
- Fiber: 2g
- Sugar: 6g
- Portion Size: 1 cup

Grilled Portobello Mushroom Burger

Ingredients:

- 4 large portobello mushrooms, stems removed
- 2 tbsp balsamic vinegar
- 1 tbsp olive oil
- 4 whole grain buns
- Lettuce leaves
- Tomato slices
- Red onion slices

Instructions:

1. Marinate mushrooms in balsamic vinegar and olive oil for 10 minutes.
2. Grill mushrooms over medium heat for 5 minutes per side.
3. Serve on buns with lettuce, tomato, and onion.

Nutrition Information (per burger):

- Calories: 250
- Protein: 8g
- Carbohydrates: 35g
- Fat: 8g
- Fiber: 5g
- Sugar: 6g
- Portion Size: 1 burger

Sweet Potato and Black Bean Tacos

Ingredients:

- 2 large sweet potatoes, peeled and diced
- 1 can (15 oz) black beans, rinsed and drained
- 1 tbsp olive oil
- 1 tsp cumin
- 1/2 tsp paprika
- Salt and pepper to taste
- Corn tortillas
- Avocado slices
- Fresh cilantro

Instructions:

1. Preheat oven to 400°F (200°C).
2. Toss sweet potatoes with olive oil, cumin, paprika, salt, and pepper.
3. Spread on a baking sheet and roast for 25-30 minutes.
4. Warm tortillas and fill with sweet potatoes, black beans, avocado, and cilantro.

Nutrition Information (per taco):

- Calories: 200
- Protein: 6g
- Carbohydrates: 35g

- Fat: 6g

- Fiber: 10g

- Sugar: 5g

- Portion Size: 1 taco

Kale and Quinoa Salad

Ingredients:

- 2 cups kale, chopped

- 1 cup cooked quinoa

- 1/4 cup sunflower seeds

- 1/4 cup dried cranberries

- 2 tbsp olive oil

- 1 tbsp apple cider vinegar

- Salt and pepper to taste

Instructions:

1. In a bowl, massage kale with olive oil and salt until tender.

2. Add quinoa, sunflower seeds, and cranberries.

3. Drizzle with apple cider vinegar and toss to combine.

Nutrition Information (per serving):

- Calories: 220

- Protein: 6g

- Carbohydrates: 30g

- Fat: 10g

- Fiber: 5g

- Sugar: 8g

- Portion Size: 1 cup

Hummus and Veggie Wrap

Ingredients:

- 1 whole grain wrap

- 1/4 cup hummus

- 1/4 cup cucumber, sliced

- 1/4 cup red bell pepper, sliced

- 1/4 cup shredded carrots

- 1/4 cup spinach

Instructions:

1. Spread hummus on the wrap.

2. Layer cucumber, bell pepper, carrots, and spinach.

3. Roll up the wrap tightly.

Nutrition Information (per wrap):

- Calories: 280

- Protein: 8g

- Carbohydrates: 40g

- Fat: 10g

- Fiber: 8g

- Sugar: 4g

- Portion Size: 1 wrap

Vegetable Paella

Ingredients:

- 1 tbsp olive oil

- 1 onion, chopped

- 2 garlic cloves, minced

- 1 red bell pepper, sliced

- 1 cup green beans, chopped

- 1 cup cherry tomatoes, halved

- 1 cup Arborio rice

- 2 cups vegetable broth

- 1/4 tsp saffron threads

- 1 tsp smoked paprika

- Salt and pepper to taste

- Lemon wedges for serving

Instructions:

1. Heat olive oil in a large pan, sauté onion and garlic until soft.

2. Add bell pepper, green beans, and cherry tomatoes, cook for
    5 minutes.

3. Stir in rice, vegetable broth, saffron, and paprika.

4. Bring to a boil, reduce heat, and simmer for 20 minutes.

5. Season with salt and pepper and serve with lemon wedges.

Nutrition Information (per serving):

- Calories: 250
- Protein: 6g
- Carbohydrates: 45g
- Fat: 6g
- Fiber: 5g
- Sugar: 5g
- Portion Size: 1 cup

Chapter 4: Dinner Recipes

Dinner is a crucial meal, especially for those managing Type 1 diabetes. A well-balanced dinner should provide enough nutrients to maintain energy levels and stabilize blood sugar through the night. The following recipes are designed to be both nutritious and delicious, perfect for anyone looking to enjoy a satisfying evening meal without compromising their health.

Eggplant Parmesan

Ingredients:

- 2 large eggplants, sliced into rounds
- 1 cup whole wheat breadcrumbs
- 1 cup grated Parmesan cheese
- 2 cups marinara sauce
- 1 ½ cups shredded mozzarella cheese
- 2 eggs, beaten
- 2 tablespoons olive oil
- Salt and pepper to taste
- Fresh basil for garnish

Instructions:

1. Preheat oven to 375°F (190°C).

2. Sprinkle eggplant slices with salt and let sit for 30 minutes. Pat dry.

3. Dip each slice into beaten eggs, then coat with breadcrumbs mixed with Parmesan.

4. Place on a baking sheet and drizzle with olive oil. Bake for 25 minutes, flipping halfway.

5. Spread a thin layer of marinara sauce in a baking dish. Layer with eggplant slices, marinara, and mozzarella. Repeat.

6. Bake for another 20 minutes until cheese is melted and bubbly. Garnish with fresh basil before serving.

Nutrition Information (per serving):

- Calories: 310
- Protein: 15g
- Carbohydrates: 30g
- Fat: 15g
- Fiber: 7g
- Sugar: 9g
- Portion Size: 1 slice

Stuffed Bell Peppers

Ingredients:

- 4 bell peppers, tops cut off and seeds removed

- 1 cup cooked quinoa

- 1 can black beans, drained and rinsed

- 1 cup corn kernels

- 1 cup diced tomatoes

- 1 teaspoon cumin

- 1 teaspoon chili powder

- 1 cup shredded cheddar cheese

- Salt and pepper to taste

- Fresh cilantro for garnish

Instructions:

1. Preheat oven to 375°F (190°C).

2. In a large bowl, mix quinoa, black beans, corn, tomatoes, cumin, chili powder, salt, and pepper.

3. Stuff each bell pepper with the quinoa mixture and place in a baking dish.

4. Top with shredded cheddar cheese.

5. Bake for 30-35 minutes until peppers are tender and cheese is melted.

6. Garnish with fresh cilantro before serving.

Nutrition Information (per serving):

- Calories: 250

- Protein: 10g

- Carbohydrates: 40g

- Fat: 8g

- Fiber: 10g

- Sugar: 8g

- Portion Size: 1 stuffed pepper

Spaghetti Squash with Marinara Sauce

Ingredients:

- 1 large spaghetti squash

- 2 cups marinara sauce

- 1 tablespoon olive oil

- 1 onion, diced

- 3 cloves garlic, minced

- 1 teaspoon dried oregano

- 1 teaspoon dried basil

- Salt and pepper to taste

- Fresh parsley for garnish

Instructions:

1. Preheat oven to 400°F (200°C).

2. Cut spaghetti squash in half lengthwise and scoop out seeds.

3. Drizzle with olive oil, season with salt and pepper, and place cut-side down on a baking sheet. Roast for 40 minutes.

4. In a saucepan, heat olive oil over medium heat. Add onion and garlic, sauté until soft.

5. Add marinara sauce, oregano, basil, salt, and pepper. Simmer for 10 minutes.

6. Scrape the spaghetti squash strands with a fork and place in a bowl. Top with marinara sauce and garnish with fresh parsley.

Nutrition Information (per serving):

- Calories: 180
- Protein: 4g
- Carbohydrates: 30g
- Fat: 7g
- Fiber: 8g
- Sugar: 12g
- Portion Size: 1 cup

Veggie Stir-Fry with Tofu

Ingredients:

- 1 block firm tofu, pressed and cubed
- 2 tablespoons soy sauce
- 1 tablespoon sesame oil
- 1 red bell pepper, sliced

- 1 yellow bell pepper, sliced

- 1 cup broccoli florets

- 1 cup snap peas

- 1 carrot, julienned

- 3 cloves garlic, minced

- 1 tablespoon grated ginger

- 1 tablespoon olive oil

- 2 tablespoons sesame seeds

- Salt and pepper to taste

Instructions:

1. In a bowl, marinate tofu with soy sauce and sesame oil for 15 minutes.

2. Heat olive oil in a large skillet over medium-high heat. Add tofu and cook until golden brown. Remove and set aside.

3. In the same skillet, add garlic and ginger, sauté for 1 minute.

4. Add bell peppers, broccoli, snap peas, and carrot. Stir-fry until tender-crisp.

5. Return tofu to the skillet and toss to combine. Season with salt and pepper.

6. Sprinkle with sesame seeds before serving.

Nutrition Information (per serving):

- Calories: 220

- Protein: 12g

- Carbohydrates: 15g

- Fat: 14g

- Fiber: 5g

- Sugar: 5g

- Portion Size: 1 cup

Cauliflower Crust Pizza

Ingredients:

- 1 head cauliflower, grated

- 1 cup shredded mozzarella cheese

- 1/4 cup grated Parmesan cheese

- 1 egg, beaten

- 1 teaspoon dried oregano

- 1 teaspoon garlic powder

- 1/2 cup marinara sauce

- 1 cup mixed vegetables (bell peppers, onions, mushrooms)

- Salt and pepper to taste

- Fresh basil for garnish

Instructions:

1. Preheat oven to 425°F (220°C). Line a baking sheet with parchment paper.

2. Microwave grated cauliflower for 8 minutes. Let cool and squeeze out excess moisture.

3. In a bowl, mix cauliflower, mozzarella, Parmesan, egg, oregano, garlic powder, salt, and pepper. Form into a crust on the baking sheet.

4. Bake for 15-20 minutes until golden.

5. Spread marinara sauce over the crust. Top with mixed vegetables and remaining mozzarella.

6. Bake for another 10 minutes until cheese is melted. Garnish with fresh basil.

Nutrition Information (per serving):

- Calories: 180
- Protein: 12g
- Carbohydrates: 10g
- Fat: 10g
- Fiber: 4g
- Sugar: 5g
- Portion Size: 1 slice

Mushroom and Spinach Lasagna

Ingredients:

- 12 whole wheat lasagna noodles

- 2 cups ricotta cheese

- 1 cup shredded mozzarella cheese

- 1/2 cup grated Parmesan cheese

- 3 cups marinara sauce

- 2 cups mushrooms, sliced

- 4 cups fresh spinach

- 1 onion, diced

- 3 cloves garlic, minced

- 1 tablespoon olive oil

- Salt and pepper to taste

Instructions:

1. Preheat oven to 375°F (190°C). Cook lasagna noodles according to package instructions.

2. In a skillet, heat olive oil over medium heat. Add onion and garlic, sauté until soft.

3. Add mushrooms and spinach, cook until wilted. Season with salt and pepper.

4. In a baking dish, spread a layer of marinara sauce. Layer with noodles, ricotta, mushroom-spinach mixture, and mozzarella. Repeat.

5. Top with Parmesan cheese.

6. Bake for 25-30 minutes until bubbly and golden.

Nutrition Information (per serving):

- Calories: 320
- Protein: 18g
- Carbohydrates: 40g
- Fat: 12g
- Fiber: 7g
- Sugar: 10g
- Portion Size: 1 piece

Sweet Potato and Lentil Curry

Ingredients:

- 2 large sweet potatoes, peeled and cubed
- 1 cup red lentils
- 1 can coconut milk
- 1 can diced tomatoes
- 1 onion, diced
- 3 cloves garlic, minced
- 1 tablespoon grated ginger
- 2 teaspoons curry powder
- 1 teaspoon ground cumin
- 1 tablespoon olive oil
- Salt and pepper to taste
- Fresh cilantro for garnish

Instructions:

1. Heat olive oil in a large pot over medium heat. Add onion, garlic, and ginger, sauté until fragrant.

2. Add sweet potatoes, lentils, curry powder, and cumin. Stir to combine.

3. Pour in coconut milk and diced tomatoes. Bring to a boil, then reduce heat and simmer for 25-30 minutes until lentils and sweet potatoes are tender.

4. Season with salt and pepper.

5. Garnish with fresh cilantro before serving.

Nutrition Information (per serving):

- Calories: 280
- Protein: 10g
- Carbohydrates: 40g
- Fat: 10g
- Fiber: 8g
- Sugar: 6g
- Portion Size: 1 cup

Baked Ziti with Vegetables

Ingredients:

- 12 ounces whole wheat ziti

- 2 cups marinara sauce

- 1 cup ricotta cheese

- 1 cup shredded mozzarella cheese

- 1/2 cup grated Parmesan cheese

- 1 zucchini, sliced

- 1 yellow squash, sliced

- 1 bell pepper, diced

- 1 onion, diced

- 3 cloves garlic, minced

- 1 tablespoon olive oil

- Salt and pepper to taste

- Fresh basil for garnish

Instructions:

1. Preheat oven to 375°F (190°C). Cook ziti according to package instructions.

2. In a skillet, heat olive oil over medium heat. Add onion and garlic, sauté until soft.

3. Add zucchini, yellow squash, and bell pepper. Cook until tender. Season with salt and pepper.

4. In a large bowl, mix cooked ziti, marinara sauce, ricotta, and sautéed vegetables.

5. Transfer to a baking dish. Top with mozzarella and Parmesan cheese.

6. Bake for 20-25 minutes until cheese is melted and bubbly. Garnish with fresh basil.

Nutrition Information (per serving):

- Calories: 350
- Protein: 18g
- Carbohydrates: 45g
- Fat: 12g
- Fiber: 8g
- Sugar: 10g
- Portion Size: 1 cup

Stuffed Acorn Squash

Ingredients:

- 2 acorn squashes, halved and seeded
- 1 cup cooked quinoa
- 1 can black beans, drained and rinsed
- 1 cup corn kernels
- 1 cup diced tomatoes
- 1 teaspoon cumin
- 1 teaspoon chili powder
- 1 cup shredded cheddar cheese
- Salt and pepper to taste

- Fresh cilantro for garnish

Instructions:

1. Preheat oven to 375°F (190°C).
2. Place acorn squash halves cut-side down on a baking sheet. Roast for 30-35 minutes until tender.
3. In a bowl, mix quinoa, black beans, corn, tomatoes, cumin, chili powder, salt, and pepper.
4. Stuff each acorn squash half with the quinoa mixture. Top with shredded cheddar cheese.
5. Bake for an additional 10 minutes until cheese is melted.
6. Garnish with fresh cilantro before serving.

Nutrition Information (per serving):
- Calories: 300
- Protein: 12g
- Carbohydrates: 50g
- Fat: 10g
- Fiber: 10g
- Sugar: 8g
- Portion Size: 1 stuffed squash half

Ratatouille

Ingredients:

- 1 eggplant, diced
- 1 zucchini, diced
- 1 yellow squash, diced
- 1 red bell pepper, diced
- 1 yellow bell pepper, diced
- 1 onion, diced
- 3 cloves garlic, minced
- 2 cups diced tomatoes
- 2 tablespoons olive oil
- 1 teaspoon dried thyme
- 1 teaspoon dried basil
- Salt and pepper to taste
- Fresh parsley for garnish

Instructions:

1. Preheat oven to 375°F (190°C).
2. In a large bowl, mix eggplant, zucchini, yellow squash, bell peppers, onion, garlic, olive oil, thyme, basil, salt, and pepper.
3. Spread vegetable mixture in a baking dish.
4. Bake for 35-40 minutes until vegetables are tender.
5. Garnish with fresh parsley before serving.

Nutrition Information (per serving):

- Calories: 180
- Protein: 4g
- Carbohydrates: 20g
- Fat: 10g
- Fiber: 6g
- Sugar: 10g
- Portion Size: 1 cup

Broccoli and Cheddar Stuffed Potatoes

Ingredients:

- 4 large russet potatoes
- 1 cup broccoli florets, steamed
- 1 cup shredded cheddar cheese
- 1/2 cup Greek yogurt
- 2 tablespoons butter
- Salt and pepper to taste
- Fresh chives for garnish

Instructions:

1. Preheat oven to 400°F (200°C). Bake potatoes for 1 hour until tender.

2. Cut a slit in each potato and scoop out the insides, leaving a thin shell.

3. In a bowl, mash the potato insides with butter, Greek yogurt, salt, and pepper. Stir in steamed broccoli and half of the cheddar cheese.

4. Stuff the mixture back into the potato shells and top with remaining cheddar cheese.

5. Bake for an additional 15 minutes until cheese is melted. Garnish with fresh chives before serving.

Nutrition Information (per serving):

- Calories: 350
- Protein: 12g
- Carbohydrates: 50g
- Fat: 12g
- Fiber: 6g
- Sugar: 4g
- Portion Size: 1 stuffed potato

Vegetable Korma

Ingredients:

- 1 cup cauliflower florets
- 1 cup diced carrots

- 1 cup green peas
- 1 cup diced potatoes
- 1 onion, diced
- 3 cloves garlic, minced
- 1 tablespoon grated ginger
- 1 can coconut milk
- 1 cup vegetable broth
- 2 tablespoons korma curry paste
- 1 tablespoon olive oil
- Salt and pepper to taste
- Fresh cilantro for garnish

Instructions:

1. Heat olive oil in a large pot over medium heat. Add onion, garlic, and ginger, sauté until fragrant.
2. Add cauliflower, carrots, peas, and potatoes. Cook for 5 minutes.
3. Stir in korma curry paste and cook for another minute.
4. Pour in coconut milk and vegetable broth. Bring to a boil, then reduce heat and simmer for 20 minutes until vegetables are tender.
5. Season with salt and pepper.
6. Garnish with fresh cilantro before serving.

Nutrition Information (per serving):

- Calories: 250

- Protein: 5g

- Carbohydrates: 30g

- Fat: 12g

- Fiber: 6g

- Sugar: 8g

- Portion Size: 1 cup

Black Bean and Corn Enchiladas

Ingredients:

- 8 whole wheat tortillas

- 1 can black beans, drained and rinsed

- 1 cup corn kernels

- 1 cup diced tomatoes

- 1 cup shredded cheddar cheese

- 1 cup enchilada sauce

- 1 onion, diced

- 3 cloves garlic, minced

- 1 tablespoon olive oil

- 1 teaspoon cumin

- 1 teaspoon chili powder

- Salt and pepper to taste

- Fresh cilantro for garnish

Instructions:

1. Preheat oven to 375°F (190°C).
2. In a skillet, heat olive oil over medium heat. Add onion and garlic, sauté until soft.
3. Add black beans, corn, tomatoes, cumin, chili powder, salt, and pepper. Cook for 5 minutes.
4. Spoon the mixture onto tortillas, roll up, and place in a baking dish.
5. Pour enchilada sauce over the tortillas and top with shredded cheddar cheese.
6. Bake for 20-25 minutes until cheese is melted and bubbly. Garnish with fresh cilantro.

Nutrition Information (per serving):

- Calories: 300
- Protein: 12g
- Carbohydrates: 45g
- Fat: 10g
- Fiber: 10g
- Sugar: 6g
- Portion Size: 1 enchilada

Grilled Vegetable Skewers

Ingredients:

- 1 red bell pepper, cut into chunks
- 1 yellow bell pepper, cut into chunks
- 1 zucchini, sliced
- 1 yellow squash, sliced
- 1 red onion, cut into chunks
- 1 cup cherry tomatoes
- 2 tablespoons olive oil
- 1 teaspoon dried oregano
- 1 teaspoon garlic powder
- Salt and pepper to taste
- Fresh basil for garnish

Instructions:

1. Preheat grill to medium-high heat.
2. In a large bowl, toss vegetables with olive oil, oregano, garlic powder, salt, and pepper.
3. Thread the vegetables onto skewers.
4. Grill for 10-15 minutes, turning occasionally, until vegetables are tender and lightly charred.
5. Garnish with fresh basil before serving.

Nutrition Information (per serving):

- Calories: 150
- Protein: 3g
- Carbohydrates: 15g
- Fat: 10g
- Fiber: 5g
- Sugar: 8g
- Portion Size: 2 skewers

Chickpea and Spinach Stew

Ingredients:

- 2 cans chickpeas, drained and rinsed
- 4 cups fresh spinach
- 1 onion, diced
- 3 cloves garlic, minced
- 1 can diced tomatoes
- 1 teaspoon ground cumin
- 1 teaspoon paprika
- 1 teaspoon ground coriander
- 2 cups vegetable broth
- 1 tablespoon olive oil
- Salt and pepper to taste
- Fresh parsley for garnish

Instructions:

1. Heat olive oil in a large pot over medium heat. Add onion and garlic, sauté until soft.
2. Add cumin, paprika, and coriander, cook for another minute.
3. Stir in chickpeas, diced tomatoes, and vegetable broth. Bring to a boil, then reduce heat and simmer for 15 minutes.
4. Add fresh spinach and cook until wilted. Season with salt and pepper.
5. Garnish with fresh parsley before serving.

Nutrition Information (per serving):

- Calories: 230
- Protein: 10g
- Carbohydrates: 30g
- Fat: 8g
- Fiber: 8g
- Sugar: 6g
- Portion Size: 1 cup

Chapter 5: Snacks and Appetizers

Eating healthy snacks and appetizers is crucial for managing Type 1 diabetes, especially when following a vegetarian diet. The right snacks can help maintain blood sugar levels, provide essential nutrients, and keep you feeling satisfied between meals.

Hummus with Veggie Sticks

Ingredients:

- 1 can chickpeas, drained and rinsed
- 2 tbsp tahini
- 1 clove garlic, minced
- Juice of 1 lemon
- 2 tbsp olive oil
- Salt to taste
- Assorted veggie sticks (carrots, celery, bell peppers, cucumbers)

Instructions:

1. In a food processor, blend chickpeas, tahini, garlic, and lemon juice until smooth.
2. Gradually add olive oil while blending until creamy.
3. Season with salt to taste.

4. Serve with assorted veggie sticks.

Nutrition Information (Per Serving):

- Calories: 150

- Protein: 5g

- Carbohydrates: 15g

- Fat: 8g

- Fiber: 4g

- Sugar: 2g

- Portion Size: 1/4 cup hummus with 1 cup veggies

Baked Kale Chips

Ingredients:

- 1 bunch kale, washed and torn into pieces

- 1 tbsp olive oil

- Salt to taste

Instructions:

1. Preheat oven to 350°F (175°C).

2. Toss kale pieces with olive oil and salt.

3. Spread on a baking sheet in a single layer.

4. Bake for 10-15 minutes until crispy.

Nutrition Information (Per Serving):

- Calories: 60
- Protein: 2g
- Carbohydrates: 7g
- Fat: 3g
- Fiber: 2g
- Sugar: 1g
- Portion Size: 1 cup

Roasted Chickpeas

Ingredients:

- 1 can chickpeas, drained and rinsed
- 1 tbsp olive oil
- 1 tsp paprika
- 1/2 tsp garlic powder
- Salt to taste

Instructions:

1. Preheat oven to 400°F (200°C).
2. Toss chickpeas with olive oil, paprika, garlic powder, and salt.
3. Spread on a baking sheet.
4. Roast for 20-25 minutes until crispy.

Nutrition Information (Per Serving):

- Calories: 120
- Protein: 5g
- Carbohydrates: 17g
- Fat: 4g
- Fiber: 5g
- Sugar: 1g
- Portion Size: 1/2 cup

Guacamole with Whole Grain Crackers

Ingredients:

- 2 ripe avocados
- 1 lime, juiced
- 1/4 cup diced red onion
- 1 small tomato, diced
- Salt and pepper to taste
- Whole grain crackers

Instructions:

1. Mash avocados in a bowl.
2. Mix in lime juice, red onion, and tomato.
3. Season with salt and pepper.
4. Serve with whole grain crackers.

Nutrition Information (Per Serving):

- Calories: 180
- Protein: 3g
- Carbohydrates: 12g
- Fat: 15g
- Fiber: 7g
- Sugar: 1g
- Portion Size: 1/4 cup guacamole with 10 crackers

Veggie Spring Rolls

Ingredients:

- 8 rice paper wrappers
- 1 cup shredded carrots
- 1 cup sliced cucumber
- 1 cup shredded lettuce
- 1/2 cup fresh mint leaves
- 1/2 cup fresh basil leaves
- Dipping sauce of choice

Instructions:

1. Soak rice paper wrappers in warm water until soft.
2. Lay on a flat surface and fill with carrots, cucumber, lettuce, mint, and basil.

3. Roll tightly and serve with dipping sauce.

Nutrition Information (Per Serving):

- Calories: 50

- Protein: 1g

- Carbohydrates: 10g

- Fat: 0g

- Fiber: 1g

- Sugar: 2g

- Portion Size: 2 rolls

Greek Yogurt Dip with Cucumber Slices

Ingredients:

- 1 cup plain Greek yogurt

- 1 tbsp fresh dill, chopped

- 1 clove garlic, minced

- 1 tbsp lemon juice

- Salt to taste

- Sliced cucumbers

Instructions:

1. Mix Greek yogurt, dill, garlic, lemon juice, and salt in a bowl.

2. Serve with cucumber slices.

Nutrition Information (Per Serving):

- Calories: 80

- Protein: 8g

- Carbohydrates: 5g

- Fat: 3g

- Fiber: 0g

- Sugar: 4g

- Portion Size: 1/4 cup dip with 1 cup cucumber slices

Stuffed Mini Peppers

Ingredients:

- 12 mini bell peppers

- 1/2 cup hummus

- 1/4 cup feta cheese, crumbled

Instructions:

1. Cut tops off mini peppers and remove seeds.

2. Fill each pepper with hummus.

3. Top with crumbled feta cheese.

Nutrition Information (Per Serving):

- Calories: 100
- Protein: 3g
- Carbohydrates: 12g
- Fat: 5g
- Fiber: 3g
- Sugar: 4g
- Portion Size: 4 stuffed peppers

Almond Butter Apple Slices

Ingredients:

- 1 apple, sliced
- 2 tbsp almond butter
- 1 tsp cinnamon

Instructions:

1. Spread almond butter on apple slices.
2. Sprinkle with cinnamon.

Nutrition Information (Per Serving):

- Calories: 150
- Protein: 2g
- Carbohydrates: 20g

- Fat: 8g
- Fiber: 4g
- Sugar: 15g
- Portion Size: 1 apple with 2 tbsp almond butter

Edamame with Sea Salt

Ingredients:

- 1 cup edamame
- Sea salt to taste

Instructions:

1. Steam edamame until tender.
2. Sprinkle with sea salt.

Nutrition Information (Per Serving):

- Calories: 120
- Protein: 11g
- Carbohydrates: 10g
- Fat: 5g
- Fiber: 5g
- Sugar: 2g
- Portion Size: 1 cup

Spicy Roasted Cauliflower Bites

Ingredients:

- 1 head cauliflower, cut into florets
- 2 tbsp olive oil
- 1 tsp paprika
- 1/2 tsp chili powder
- Salt to taste

Instructions:

1. Preheat oven to 400°F (200°C).
2. Toss cauliflower florets with olive oil, paprika, chili powder, and salt.
3. Spread on a baking sheet.
4. Roast for 25-30 minutes until tender.

Nutrition Information (Per Serving):

- Calories: 80
- Protein: 2g
- Carbohydrates: 8g
- Fat: 5g
- Fiber: 3g
- Sugar: 2g
- Portion Size: 1 cup

Caprese Skewers

Ingredients:

- 1 pint cherry tomatoes
- 8 oz mozzarella balls
- Fresh basil leaves
- Balsamic glaze

Instructions:

1. Thread cherry tomatoes, mozzarella balls, and basil leaves onto skewers.
2. Drizzle with balsamic glaze.

Nutrition Information (Per Serving):

- Calories: 100
- Protein: 5g
- Carbohydrates: 4g
- Fat: 6g
- Fiber: 1g
- Sugar: 2g
- Portion Size: 4 skewers

Veggie Sushi Rolls

Ingredients:

- 1 cup sushi rice, cooked
- 1 cucumber, julienned
- 1 carrot, julienned
- 1 avocado, sliced
- Nori sheets

Instructions:

1. Spread a thin layer of rice on a nori sheet.
2. Place cucumber, carrot, and avocado in the center.
3. Roll tightly and slice into pieces.

Nutrition Information (Per Serving):

- Calories: 120
- Protein: 2g
- Carbohydrates: 22g
- Fat: 3g
- Fiber: 3g
- Sugar: 1g
- Portion Size: 1 roll

Parmesan Zucchini Fries

Ingredients:

- 2 medium zucchinis
- 1/2 cup grated Parmesan cheese
- 1/2 teaspoon garlic powder
- 1/2 teaspoon dried oregano
- Salt and pepper to taste

Instructions:

1. Preheat the oven to 425°F (220°C). Line a baking sheet with parchment paper.
2. Cut the zucchinis into sticks resembling fries.
3. In a bowl, combine Parmesan cheese, garlic powder, dried oregano, salt, and pepper.
4. Coat each zucchini stick with the Parmesan mixture.
5. Place the coated zucchini sticks on the baking sheet in a single layer.
6. Bake for 20-25 minutes or until golden and crispy.
7. Serve hot.

Nutrition Information:

- Calories: 120
- Protein: 8g
- Carbohydrates: 10g

- Fat: 6g

- Fiber: 3g

- Sugar: 5g

- Portion Size: 1 serving

Mini Quiche Cups

Ingredients:

- 4 large eggs

- 1/2 cup milk or almond milk

- 1/2 cup grated cheese (cheddar or Swiss)

- 1/2 cup diced vegetables (spinach, bell peppers, onions)

- Salt and pepper to taste

Instructions:

1. Preheat the oven to 350°F (175°C). Grease a muffin tin or line with paper liners.

2. In a bowl, whisk together eggs, milk, salt, and pepper.

3. Stir in grated cheese and diced vegetables.

4. Pour the egg mixture evenly into the muffin cups.

5. Bake for 20-25 minutes or until the quiches are set and golden on top.

6. Let cool slightly before serving.

Nutrition Information:

- Calories: 100
- Protein: 7g
- Carbohydrates: 3g
- Fat: 6g
- Fiber: 1g
- Sugar: 2g
- Portion Size: 2 mini quiche cups

Berry and Nut Mix

Ingredients:

- 1/2 cup almonds
- 1/2 cup walnuts
- 1/2 cup dried cranberries
- 1/2 cup dried blueberries

Instructions:

1. Mix all ingredients together in a bowl.
2. Store in an airtight container.
3. Enjoy as a quick and nutritious snack.

Nutrition Information:

- Calories: 160

- Protein: 5g

- Carbohydrates: 15g

- Fat: 10g

- Fiber: 3g

- Sugar: 9g

- Portion Size: 1/4 cup

Chapter 6: Desserts

Desserts are the delightful conclusion to any meal, offering a sweet end to your culinary journey. This chapter presents a collection of delectable desserts that range from rich chocolate treats to refreshing fruit-based delights. Each recipe is designed to satisfy your sweet tooth while providing a balance of nutrients. Enjoy these desserts knowing that they are crafted with health in mind.

Chia Seed Pudding with Mango

Ingredients:

- 1/4 cup chia seeds
- 1 cup almond milk
- 1 tbsp maple syrup
- 1 tsp vanilla extract
- 1 ripe mango, diced

Instructions:

1. Mix chia seeds, almond milk, maple syrup, and vanilla extract in a bowl.
2. Refrigerate for at least 2 hours or overnight.
3. Top with diced mango before serving.

Nutrition Information (per serving):

- Calories: 200
- Protein: 4g
- Carbohydrates: 30g
- Fat: 8g
- Fiber: 8g
- Sugar: 18g
- Portion Size: 1 cup

Chocolate Avocado Mousse

Ingredients:

- 2 ripe avocados
- 1/4 cup cocoa powder
- 1/4 cup almond milk
- 1/4 cup honey or maple syrup
- 1 tsp vanilla extract

Instructions:

1. Blend all ingredients until smooth.
2. Refrigerate for 30 minutes before serving.

Nutrition Information (per serving):

- Calories: 250

- Protein: 3g

- Carbohydrates: 30g

- Fat: 15g

- Fiber: 8g

- Sugar: 20g

- Portion Size: 1/2 cup

Baked Apples with Cinnamon

Ingredients:

- 4 apples

- 2 tbsp maple syrup

- 1 tsp cinnamon

- 1/4 cup chopped walnuts

Instructions:

1. Core the apples and place them in a baking dish.

2. Drizzle with maple syrup and sprinkle with cinnamon and walnuts.

3. Bake at 350°F (175°C) for 20-25 minutes.

Nutrition Information (per serving):

- Calories: 150

- Protein: 1g

- Carbohydrates: 25g
- Fat: 5g
- Fiber: 4g
- Sugar: 18g
- Portion Size: 1 apple

Greek Yogurt Parfait with Berries

Ingredients:

- 1 cup Greek yogurt
- 1/2 cup mixed berries
- 2 tbsp granola
- 1 tbsp honey

Instructions:

1. Layer Greek yogurt, mixed berries, and granola in a glass.
2. Drizzle with honey.

Nutrition Information (per serving):

- Calories: 200
- Protein: 10g
- Carbohydrates: 30g
- Fat: 5g
- Fiber: 4g

- Sugar: 20g
- Portion Size: 1 cup

Almond Flour Brownies

Ingredients:

- 1 cup almond flour
- 1/2 cup cocoa powder
- 1/2 cup maple syrup
- 1/4 cup coconut oil, melted
- 2 eggs
- 1 tsp vanilla extract

Instructions:

1. Mix all ingredients until well combined.
2. Pour into a greased baking dish and bake at 350°F (175°C) for 20-25 minutes.

Nutrition Information (per serving):

- Calories: 200
- Protein: 4g
- Carbohydrates: 20g
- Fat: 12g
- Fiber: 3g

- Sugar: 14g
- Portion Size: 1 brownie

Banana Ice Cream

Ingredients:

- 2 ripe bananas, sliced and frozen
- 1 tsp vanilla extract
- 2 tbsp almond milk

Instructions:

1. Blend all ingredients until smooth.
2. Serve immediately or freeze for a firmer texture.

Nutrition Information (per serving):

- Calories: 150
- Protein: 2g
- Carbohydrates: 35g
- Fat: 1g
- Fiber: 4g
- Sugar: 20g
- Portion Size: 1 cup

Carrot Cake Energy Balls

Ingredients:

- 1 cup shredded carrots
- 1 cup rolled oats
- 1/2 cup almond butter
- 1/4 cup honey
- 1 tsp cinnamon

Instructions:

1. Mix all ingredients until well combined.
2. Roll into balls and refrigerate for at least 30 minutes.

Nutrition Information (per serving):

- Calories: 100
- Protein: 3g
- Carbohydrates: 12g
- Fat: 5g
- Fiber: 2g
- Sugar: 6g
- Portion Size: 2 balls

Strawberry Chia Jam Bars

Ingredients:

- 1 cup strawberries, mashed
- 2 tbsp chia seeds
- 1 tbsp honey
- 1 cup almond flour
- 1/4 cup coconut oil, melted
- 1/4 cup honey

Instructions:

1. Mix strawberries, chia seeds, and honey; refrigerate until set.
2. Combine almond flour, coconut oil, and honey; press into a baking dish.
3. Spread the jam over the base and bake at 350°F (175°C) for 15-20 minutes.

Nutrition Information (per serving):

- Calories: 180
- Protein: 3g
- Carbohydrates: 20g
- Fat: 10g
- Fiber: 4g
- Sugar: 12g
- Portion Size: 1 bar

Apple Cinnamon Muffins

Ingredients:

- 1 cup whole wheat flour
- 1/2 cup rolled oats
- 1 tsp baking powder
- 1 tsp cinnamon
- 1/2 cup applesauce
- 1/4 cup honey
- 1/4 cup almond milk
- 1 apple, diced

Instructions:

1. Mix dry and wet ingredients separately, then combine.
2. Fold in diced apple and spoon into muffin tin.
3. Bake at 350°F (175°C) for 20-25 minutes.

Nutrition Information (per serving):

- Calories: 150
- Protein: 3g
- Carbohydrates: 30g
- Fat: 2g
- Fiber: 4g
- Sugar: 12g
- Portion Size: 1 muffin

Blueberry Crumble

Ingredients:

- 2 cups blueberries
- 1 tbsp honey
- 1 cup rolled oats
- 1/4 cup almond flour
- 1/4 cup coconut oil, melted
- 1/4 cup honey

Instructions:

1. Mix blueberries and honey, place in a baking dish.
2. Combine oats, almond flour, coconut oil, and honey; spread over blueberries.
3. Bake at 350°F (175°C) for 25-30 minutes.

Nutrition Information (per serving):

- Calories: 200
- Protein: 3g
- Carbohydrates: 30g
- Fat: 8g
- Fiber: 5g
- Sugar: 18g
- Portion Size: 1/2 cup

Coconut Macaroons

Ingredients:

- 2 cups shredded coconut
- 1/4 cup honey
- 2 egg whites
- 1 tsp vanilla extract

Instructions:

1. Mix all ingredients until well combined.
2. Scoop onto a baking sheet and bake at 350°F (175°C) for 15-20 minutes.

Nutrition Information (per serving):

- Calories: 150
- Protein: 2g
- Carbohydrates: 15g
- Fat: 10g
- Fiber: 3g
- Sugar: 12g
- Portion Size: 2 macaroons

Dark Chocolate Covered Almonds

Ingredients:

- 1 cup almonds
- 1/2 cup dark chocolate, melted
- 1/2 tsp sea salt

Instructions:

1. Dip almonds in melted chocolate.
2. Spread on parchment paper and sprinkle with sea salt.
3. Let cool until chocolate sets.

Nutrition Information (per serving):

- Calories: 200
- Protein: 5g
- Carbohydrates: 15g
- Fat: 15g
- Fiber: 4g
- Sugar: 10g
- Portion Size: 1/4 cup

Pumpkin Pie Bites

Ingredients:

- 1 cup canned pumpkin

- 1/4 cup almond flour
- 1/4 cup maple syrup
- 1 tsp pumpkin pie spice

Instructions:

1. Mix all ingredients until well combined.
2. Spoon into a mini muffin tin and bake at 350°F (175°C) for 15-20 minutes.

Nutrition Information (per serving):

- Calories: 100
- Protein: 2g
- Carbohydrates: 15g
- Fat: 4g
- Fiber: 2g
- Sugar: 8g
- Portion Size: 2 bites

Lemon Yogurt Popsicles

Ingredients:

- 1 cup Greek yogurt
- 1/4 cup lemon juice
- 1/4 cup honey

- 1 tsp lemon zest

Instructions:

1. Mix all ingredients until smooth.
2. Pour into popsicle molds and freeze until solid.

Nutrition Information (per serving):

- Calories: 100
- Protein: 5g
- Carbohydrates: 18g
- Fat: 1g
- Fiber: 0g
- Sugar: 15g
- Portion Size: 1 popsicle

Mixed Berry Sorbet

Ingredients:

- 2 cups mixed berries, frozen
- 1/4 cup honey
- 1/4 cup water

Instructions:

1. Blend all ingredients until smooth.

2. Freeze for 1-2 hours before serving.

Nutrition Information (per serving):

- Calories: 100

- Protein: 1g

- Carbohydrates: 25g

- Fat: 0g

- Fiber: 4g

- Sugar: 20g

- Portion Size: 1/2 cup

Chapter 7: Smoothies

Smoothies are an excellent way to incorporate more fruits and vegetables into your diet. They can serve as a quick breakfast, a nutritious snack, or a post-workout refuel. The following smoothie recipes are packed with vitamins, minerals, and antioxidants, ensuring that you enjoy both taste and health benefits in every sip.

Green Detox Smoothie

Ingredients:

- 1 cup spinach
- 1/2 cucumber
- 1 green apple, cored and chopped
- 1/2 lemon, juiced
- 1/2 cup water
- 1/2 cup ice

Instructions:

1. Add all ingredients to a blender.
2. Blend until smooth.
3. Pour into a glass and serve immediately.

Nutrition Information (per serving):

- Calories: 60
- Protein: 1g
- Carbohydrates: 14g
- Fat: 0g
- Fiber: 3g
- Sugar: 8g
- Portion Size: 1 cup

Berry Blast Smoothie

Ingredients:

- 1 cup mixed berries (strawberries, blueberries, raspberries)
- 1/2 banana
- 1/2 cup Greek yogurt
- 1/2 cup almond milk
- 1 tablespoon honey

Instructions:

1. Combine all ingredients in a blender.
2. Blend until smooth.
3. Serve chilled.

Nutrition Information (per serving):

- Calories: 150
- Protein: 5g
- Carbohydrates: 30g
- Fat: 2g
- Fiber: 4g
- Sugar: 20g
- Portion Size: 1 cup

Tropical Mango Smoothie

Ingredients:

- 1 cup mango chunks
- 1/2 cup pineapple chunks
- 1/2 banana
- 1/2 cup coconut water
- 1/2 cup ice

Instructions:

1. Blend all ingredients until smooth.
2. Pour into a glass and enjoy.

Nutrition Information (per serving):

- Calories: 130

- Protein: 1g

- Carbohydrates: 33g

- Fat: 0g

- Fiber: 3g

- Sugar: 28g

- Portion Size: 1 cup

Spinach and Avocado Smoothie

Ingredients:

- 1 cup spinach

- 1/2 avocado

- 1/2 banana

- 1/2 cup almond milk

- 1 tablespoon chia seeds

Instructions:

1. Place all ingredients in a blender.

2. Blend until creamy.

3. Serve immediately.

Nutrition Information (per serving):

- Calories: 180

- Protein: 3g

- Carbohydrates: 20g

- Fat: 12g

- Fiber: 7g

- Sugar: 8g

- Portion Size: 1 cup

Peanut Butter Banana Smoothie

Ingredients:

- 1 banana

- 1 tablespoon peanut butter

- 1/2 cup Greek yogurt

- 1/2 cup almond milk

- 1 teaspoon honey

Instructions:

1. Blend all ingredients until smooth.

2. Enjoy immediately.

Nutrition Information (per serving):

- Calories: 250

- Protein: 10g

- Carbohydrates: 35g

- Fat: 10g

- Fiber: 3g

- Sugar: 20g

- Portion Size: 1 cup

Chocolate Protein Smoothie

Ingredients:

- 1 scoop chocolate protein powder

- 1 banana

- 1 tablespoon cocoa powder

- 1/2 cup almond milk

- 1/2 cup ice

Instructions:

1. Combine all ingredients in a blender.

2. Blend until smooth.

3. Serve chilled.

Nutrition Information (per serving):

- Calories: 220

- Protein: 20g

- Carbohydrates: 30g

- Fat: 4g

- Fiber: 5g

- Sugar: 15g
- Portion Size: 1 cup

Pineapple Kale Smoothie

Ingredients:

- 1 cup kale
- 1/2 cup pineapple chunks
- 1/2 banana
- 1/2 cup orange juice
- 1/2 cup ice

Instructions:

1. Blend all ingredients until smooth.
2. Enjoy immediately.

Nutrition Information (per serving):

- Calories: 110
- Protein: 2g
- Carbohydrates: 25g
- Fat: 0g
- Fiber: 3g
- Sugar: 20g
- Portion Size: 1 cup

Beetroot and Berry Smoothie

Ingredients:

- 1 small beetroot, cooked and chopped
- 1/2 cup mixed berries
- 1/2 cup Greek yogurt
- 1/2 cup water
- 1 tablespoon honey

Instructions:

1. Blend all ingredients until smooth.
2. Serve immediately.

Nutrition Information (per serving):

- Calories: 140
- Protein: 4g
- Carbohydrates: 30g
- Fat: 1g
- Fiber: 5g
- Sugar: 20g
- Portion Size: 1 cup

Carrot Ginger Smoothie

Ingredients:

- 1 cup carrot juice
- 1/2 banana
- 1/2 inch ginger, peeled
- 1/2 cup Greek yogurt
- 1 tablespoon honey

Instructions:

1. Blend all ingredients until smooth.
2. Pour into a glass and enjoy.

Nutrition Information (per serving):

- Calories: 130
- Protein: 4g
- Carbohydrates: 28g
- Fat: 1g
- Fiber: 3g
- Sugar: 20g
- Portion Size: 1 cup

Apple Pie Smoothie

Ingredients:

- 1 apple, cored and chopped
- 1/2 cup Greek yogurt
- 1/2 cup almond milk
- 1 teaspoon cinnamon
- 1 tablespoon honey

Instructions:

1. Blend all ingredients until smooth.
2. Serve chilled.

Nutrition Information (per serving):

- Calories: 150
- Protein: 4g
- Carbohydrates: 30g
- Fat: 2g
- Fiber: 4g
- Sugar: 20g
- Portion Size: 1 cup

Citrus Sunshine Smoothie

Ingredients:

- 1 orange, peeled and segmented
- 1/2 grapefruit, peeled and segmented
- 1/2 banana
- 1/2 cup coconut water
- 1 tablespoon honey

Instructions:

1. Blend all ingredients until smooth.
2. Serve immediately.

Nutrition Information (per serving):

- Calories: 130
- Protein: 1g
- Carbohydrates: 30g
- Fat: 0g
- Fiber: 3g
- Sugar: 25g
- Portion Size: 1 cup

Strawberry Banana Smoothie

Ingredients:

- 1 cup strawberries
- 1/2 banana
- 1/2 cup Greek yogurt
- 1/2 cup almond milk
- 1 tablespoon honey

Instructions:

1. Blend all ingredients until smooth.
2. Serve chilled.

Nutrition Information (per serving):

- Calories: 150
- Protein: 4g
- Carbohydrates: 30g
- Fat: 2g
- Fiber: 3g
- Sugar: 20g
- Portion Size: 1 cup

Matcha Green Tea Smoothie

Ingredients:

- 1 teaspoon matcha powder
- 1/2 banana
- 1/2 cup Greek yogurt
- 1/2 cup almond milk
- 1 tablespoon honey

Instructions:

1. Blend all ingredients until smooth.
2. Pour into a glass and enjoy.

Nutrition Information (per serving):

- Calories: 140
- Protein: 5g
- Carbohydrates: 25g
- Fat: 2g
- Fiber: 2g
- Sugar: 18g
- Portion Size: 1 cup

Watermelon Mint Smoothie

Ingredients:

- 1 cup watermelon chunks
- 1/2 cucumber
- 1 tablespoon fresh mint leaves
- 1/2 cup water
- 1/2 cup ice

Instructions:

1. Blend all ingredients until smooth.
2. Serve immediately.

Nutrition Information (per serving):

- Calories: 50
- Protein: 1g
- Carbohydrates: 12g
- Fat: 0g
- Fiber: 1g
- Sugar: 10g
- Portion Size: 1 cup

Chia Seed Power Smoothie

Ingredients:

- 1 tablespoon chia seeds
- 1/2 banana
- 1/2 cup mixed berries
- 1/2 cup almond milk
- 1 tablespoon honey

Instructions:

1. Combine all ingredients in a blender.
2. Blend until smooth.
3. Serve chilled.

Nutrition Information (per serving):

- Calories: 150
- Protein: 3g
- Carbohydrates: 30g
- Fat: 3g
- Fiber: 6g
- Sugar: 20g
- Portion Size: 1 cup

CONCLUSION

Congratulations on completing the journey through the "Diabetic Type 1 Vegetarian Cookbook for Beginners"! This book was crafted with the utmost care to empower you on your path to managing Type 1 diabetes through delicious and nourishing vegetarian meals.

Throughout these pages, you've explored a variety of recipes designed to support stable blood sugar levels while delighting your taste buds. From hearty breakfasts to satisfying dinners, energizing smoothies to guilt-free desserts, each recipe has been thoughtfully curated to balance nutrition with flavor.

As you conclude this book, remember that your journey towards better health is a continuous one. Embrace the principles of mindful eating, incorporate these recipes into your routine, and discover the joy of preparing meals that not only support your health but also bring joy to your table.

Always remember, you have the power to take charge of your health through your food choices. With a foundation of nutritious vegetarian dishes, equipped with the knowledge and inspiration from this cookbook, you are well-prepared to navigate your diabetic journey with confidence and creativity.

Here's to your health, wellness, and culinary adventures ahead!

www.ingramcontent.com/pod-product-compliance
Lightning Source LLC
Chambersburg PA
CBHW072248260726
48659CB00004BA/1474